Contents

Donna's Story

When Donna was diagnosed with cancer, she was determined to beat it. She had heard about the power of smoothies and decided to give them a try.

At first, Donna was skeptical. She had tried other diets and remedies before and had yet to see any results. But after a few weeks of drinking smoothies every day, Donna started to see a difference.

Her energy levels increased and her pain and fatigue decreased. She was able to stay active and even started to enjoy exercising.

After several months of drinking smoothies, Donna's cancer symptoms had significantly decreased. Her oncologist was amazed by her progress and said that the smoothies were likely responsible for her improved health.

Donna was so relieved to have her cancer symptoms under control. And she was grateful to have discovered the power of smoothies. She knew that she would continue to drink smoothies every day to keep her cancer symptoms in check.

Donna's story is a perfect example of the power of smoothies. If you are looking for a way to reduce your cancer symptoms, then give smoothies a try. With their nutrient-rich ingredients, smoothies can help

you stay healthy and feel your best.

Anti Cancer smoothie.

A smoothie is a drink made from pureed raw fruit and/or vegetables, typically using a blender. A smoothie often has a liquid base such as water, fruit juice, plant milk, and sometimes dairy products, such as milk, yogurt, ice cream or cottage cheese. Smoothies may be made using other ingredients, such as crushed ice, sweeteners (honey or sugar), vinegar, whey powder, chocolate or nutritional supplements, among others by personal choice. As products typically using raw fruits or vegetables, smoothies include dietary fiber (e.g. pulp, skin, and seeds) and so are thicker than fruit juice, often with a consistency similar to a milkshake. Smoothies, particularly "green smoothies" that include vegetables, may be marketed to health-conscious people for being healthier than milkshakes. The healthfulness of a smoothie depends on its ingredients and their proportions. Many smoothies include large or multiple servings of fruits and vegetables, which are recommended in a healthy diet and intended to be a meal replacement. However, fruit juice containing high amounts of sugar can increase caloric intake and promote weight gain. Similarly, ingredients such as protein powders, sweeteners, or ice cream are often used in smoothie recipes, some of which contribute mostly to flavor and further caloric intake. The most basic smoothie starts with two essential ingredients — a base and a liquid. From there, you can combine ingredients to your liking. Many smoothies include frozen produce or ice cubes to give the final product the cool, icy consistency of a milkshake. However, their flavor profiles vary tremendously depending on the ingredients.

Green smoothie

A green smoothie typically consists of 40–50% green vegetables (roughly half), usually raw green leafy vegetables, such as spinach, kale, swiss chard, collard greens, celery, parsley, or broccoli, with the remaining ingredients being mostly or entirely fruit. Wheatgrass and spirulina are also used as healthful ingredients. Most green leafy vegetables have a bitter flavor when served raw, but this can be ameliorated by choosing certain less-bitter vegetables (e.g. baby spinach) or combining with certain fruit (e.g. banana softens both the flavor and texture). Some blender manufacturers now specifically target their products towards making green smoothies and provide a booklet of recipes for them. If the fruit ingredients and the green vegetable ingredients are both juiced ahead of time, the mixed juice doesn't even have to be blended like a smoothie, i.e. a green juice. Smoothies are thick, creamy beverages usually blended from puréed fruits, vegetables, juices, yogurt, nuts, seeds, and/or dairy or nondairy milk.

☐ Common ingredients

Popular ingredients in homemade and store-bought smoothies include:

☐ Fruits: berries, banana, apple, peach, mango, and pineapple

☐ Vegetables: kale, spinach, arugula, wheatgrass, microgreens, avocado, cucumber, beetroot, cauliflower, and carrots

☐ Nuts and seeds: almond butter, peanut butter, walnut butter, sunflower seed butter, chia seeds, hemp seeds, and flax meal

☐ Herbs and spices: ginger, turmeric, cinnamon, cocoa powder, cacao nibs, parsley, and basil

☐ Nutritional and herbal supplements: spirulina, bee pollen, matcha powder, protein powder, and powdered vitamin or mineral supplements

☐ Liquid: water, fruit juice, vegetable juice, milk, nondairy milk, coconut water, iced tea, and cold brew coffee

☐ Sweeteners: maple syrup, raw sugar, honey, pitted dates, simple syrup, fruit juice concentrates, stevia, ice cream, and sorbet

☐ Others: cottage cheese, vanilla extract, soaked oats, cooked white beans, silken tofu, and dairy or nondairy yogurt

☐ Types

Most smoothies can be classified into one or two of the following categories — though there's significant overlap between them:

☐ **Fruit smoothies.**

As the name implies, this kind of smoothie usually features one or more types of fruit blended with fruit juice, water, milk, or ice cream.

☐ **Green smoothies.**

Green smoothies pack leafy green vegetables and fruit blended with water, juice, or milk. They tend to be heavier in veggies than regular smoothies, though they often include a little fruit for sweetness.

☐ **Protein smoothies.**

Protein smoothies usually start with one fruit or vegetable and a liquid, as well as a major protein source like Greek yogurt, cottage cheese, silken tofu, or protein powder. Because smoothies are so customizable, it's fairly easy to pack them with nutrients.

Smoothies are made by blending fruit, vegetables, yogurt, and other ingredients to make a thick, creamy beverage.

☐ **Potential health benefits**

Many people consume smoothies as a morning meal or afternoon snack. They can be a great way to incorporate more healthy foods into your diet.

☐ May help boost fruit and vegetable intake

Smoothies made primarily from fresh or frozen produce may increase your consumption of fruits and vegetables, which provide a diverse array of essential vitamins, minerals, fiber, and antioxidants.

☐ These nutrients may reduce inflammation, improve digestion, and lower your risk of chronic conditions like heart disease, osteoporosis, obesity, and age-related mental decline.

The World Health Organization (WHO) recommends that adults eat at least 5 servings (around 400 grams) of fruits and vegetables per day. However, most people fall short of this mark. If you find you're not eating enough fruits or veggies, a smoothie can be a delicious way to pack in 2–3 more servings.

☐ May support increased fiber consumption

Fiber is an important nutrient that aids digestion by preventing constipation and supporting the growth of beneficial bacteria in your digestive tract. Early research suggests that a healthy, thriving community of gut bacteria can help reduce inflammation, promote healthy immune function, and support mental health. Adequate fiber intake is also linked to a reduced risk of chronic illnesses, such as heart disease and type 2 diabetes. Yet, many people are not meeting their daily fiber needs — especially those who follow Western diets. The U.S. Department of Agriculture (USDA) recommends a daily intake of at least 38 grams of fiber for men and 25 grams for women. Research indicates that most Americans, on average, eat only 16 grams of fiber each day. With the right ingredients, smoothies can be an excellent way to boost your fiber intake. Some of the most fiber-rich foods are also common smoothie ingredients, including fruits, vegetables, whole grains (such as soaked oats), nuts, seeds, and legumes (such as white beans).

Some varieties contain large quantities of added sugar

The difference between a healthy and unhealthy smoothie largely depends on the quality and quantity of its ingredients. Smoothies' biggest pitfall is their propensity to contain large quantities of added sugar. Added sugar reduces the nutrient density of smoothies. Furthermore, routinely consuming too much added sugar may increase your risk of chronic ailments like heart disease, diabetes, and liver disease. The American Heart Association recommends limiting your intake of added sugar to no more than 9 teaspoons (37.5 grams) per day for men and 6 teaspoons (25 grams) per day for women (5Trusted Source). Commercially prepared smoothies tend to be higher in added sugar than homemade versions, but it ultimately depends on the ingredients used in each recipe.

For instance, Smoothie King's 20-ounce (590-mL) The Hulk Vanilla Smoothie packs 47 grams of added sugar, which is well above your daily sugar recommendation. Their Original High Protein Pineapple Smoothie is a much better option, as it provides only 4 grams of added sugar in the same serving size. Many sugary ingredients are easy to identify, such as granulated sugar, honey, maple syrup, ice cream, sherbet, and agave nectar. Nonetheless, you should keep in mind that nut butters, protein powder, flavored yogurt, fruit-flavored sauces, and sugar-sweetened juices and nondairy milks are all potential sources of added sugar.

Occasionally indulging in small quantities of added sugar is not likely harmful, but if you drink smoothies frequently, it may be best to limit sugary ingredients as much as possible. When making smoothies at home, use whole fruits, such as a ripe banana, to add sweetness instead of honey or maple syrup. When buying premade smoothies, try to limit or avoid added sugar, mainly focusing on smoothies that include whole foods like fruits and veggies. For bottled smoothies, you can find the added sugar content on the label. For made-to-order ones, check the company website or ask for nutrient information at the counter.

☐ Do smoothies aid weight loss?

Smoothies are frequently marketed as a weight loss tool. Research suggests they may be effective for this purpose as long as they're not causing you to exceed your daily calorie needs. While some people find smoothies an easy way to monitor food portions and stay on top of their weight loss goals, others may not feel as full when they drink their calories rather than eating them. That said, several small studies demonstrate that smoothies used as meal replacements can be as filling as solid foods, and that drinking calories instead of chewing them doesn't necessarily lead to overeating when solid foods are consumed later. Drinking versus chewing's effect on your feelings of fullness may be more closely related to how satisfying you expect the meal to be rather than the form of the food itself. One small study found that people who viewed a large serving of fruit prior to drinking a fruit smoothie felt fuller and more satisfied afterward, compared with people who viewed a small serving of fruit prior to drinking the smoothie. This occurred even though both groups consumed an equal amount of calories and nutrients from the smoothie.

Ultimately, although weight loss can be a complex process with many contributing factors, it's important to expend more calories than you take in. If a smoothie helps you offset other calories you would otherwise consume, it can be an effective weight loss tool. If you prioritize ingredients low in calories and high in protein and fiber, your smoothie may keep you full until your next meal. Whole fruit, vegetables, nut butters, and low or no-added-sugar yogurts are all excellent weight-loss-friendly ingredients. Keep in mind that your nutritional needs and ability to lose weight vary depending on many factors, including age, activity level, medical history, and lifestyle habits.

☐ Smoothies can be tailored to meet your needs

You can drink smoothies as a snack or meal replacement, but it's a good idea to know which types to choose — especially if you have a specific fitness or body composition goal in mind. There's a common misconception that smoothies are inherently low calorie snacks, but some smoothies pack over 1,000 calories depending on their size and ingredients. Generally, a 200–300-calorie smoothie with 10 grams of protein is a great snack, whereas a 400–800-calorie smoothie providing at least 20 grams of protein is better suited as a meal replacement. It's best to assess your goals and calorie needs to determine your specific needs. The difference between the two may be as simple as adjusting the serving size. Many smoothie chains provide the ingredient and nutrition information for each of their products, which usually come in 16–

32-ounce (475–945-mL) servings. When making smoothies at home, be sure to control your portion size. Fats like nuts, seeds, nut butters, full fat yogurts, and avocado will provide more calories but increase nutrient density. Meanwhile, sugary add-ins like syrups will provide more calories without quality nutrients.

☐ **Healthy smoothies recipes**

The most nutritious smoothies utilize whole foods, contain little or no added sugar, and include a balanced amount of carbs, fiber, protein, and healthy fats. If you want to try making smoothies at home, here are two sample recipes to get you started.

☐ **Ginger green smoothie**

Ingredients

☐ 2 cups (56 grams) of fresh baby spinach

☐ 1 large ripe banana, sliced and frozen

☐ 1 tablespoon (6 grams) of fresh ginger, roughly chopped

☐ 2 tablespoons (32 grams) of unsweetened almond butter

☐ 1/4 of a small avocado

☐ 4–6 ounces (120–180 mL) of unsweetened almond milk

☐ 1/2 cup (125 grams) of low or nonfat vanilla Greek yogurt

- Instructions

Add all ingredients to the blender and blend until smooth. If it's too thick, add more almond milk.

This recipe makes approximately 20 ounces (590 mL) and provides Calories: 513, Fat: 25 grams, Total carbs: 56 grams, Fiber: 10 grams, Added sugars: 6 grams, Protein: 21 grams.

☐ Tropical berry beet smoothie

Ingredients

☐ 1 cup (197 grams) of frozen mixed berries

☐ 1/2 cup (82 grams) of frozen mango

☐ 1/4 cup (34 grams) of raw beets, roughly chopped or grated

☐ 2 tablespoons (20 grams) of hemp hearts

☐ 1/2 cup (125 grams) of low fat plain Greek yogurt

☐ 4–6 ounces (120–180 mL) of unsweetened coconut water

☐ a squeeze of fresh lime juice

- Instructions

Add all ingredients to your blender and blend until smooth. If you want it a little sweeter, use lightly sweetened yogurt or swap the coconut water for 100% fruit juice.

This recipe makes approximately 20 ounces (590 mL) and provides Calories: 380, Fat: 13 grams, Total carbs: 52 grams, Added sugars: 0 grams, Fiber: 8 grams, Protein: 22 grams.

When making smoothies at home, aim to include a balanced combination of carbs, fiber, protein, and healthy fats. Smoothies are popular meals and snacks and can suit almost any taste or dietary preference. Their healthiness is largely determined by their ingredients. The most nutritious smoothies are made with whole foods like fruits, vegetables, yogurt, and healthy fats, while those with lots of added sugars aren't as nutrient-dense and may contribute to negative health effects over time. Smoothies high in protein and fiber may even aid weight loss by keeping you full. If you're looking for a creative way to boost your fruit and veggie intake, smoothies may be the way to go.

☐ Why smoothies are good while undergoing cancer treatment

Loss of appetite is extremely common among those fighting cancer. Not only do some types of cancer cause appetite loss themselves, but common treatments also reduce appetite as part of their side effects. Furthermore, some people may complain of sensitivity to certain smells or textures that turn them off of food. Smoothies can be a good way to partially overcome that challenge and still ensure proper nutrition. That being said, it can be easy to get into a smoothie rut. We've scoured the internet to bring you a list of five smoothies to add to your rotation. Be sure to talk to your medical team about whether or not fresh fruits and veggies are a good option for you if you happen to have a low white blood cell count!

☐ **Banana Almond Butter Smoothie**

This smoothie recipe from Real Simple Good combines four simple ingredients to create a delicious smoothie that is great as-is or that can easily be combined with your other favorite ingredients for a custom smoothie masterpiece. This recipe calls for bananas, which are a great source of fiber and potassium, as well as almond butter – a great source of protein and fat when you aren't feeling up to a steak dinner. Rounded out with coconut milk (another good source of fat) and cinnamon, we'd be surprised if this smoothie doesn't quickly become one of your favorites.

☐ **Carrot Ginger Turmeric Smoothie**

The anti-inflammatory properties of ginger and turmeric combined with carotenoid-rich carrots make Minimalist Baker's smoothie recipea slam dunk, particularly if you've been dealing with nausea. Most of the ingredients in this smoothie are also great for fortifying your immune system ... And it looks so pretty!

□ **High-Fiber Broccoli Smoothie for Kids**

Okay, this smoothie proclaims to be specifically for kids. But don't rule it out if you happen to be an adult. If there's one thing I know to be true, it's that recipes targeted for kids typically taste 300% better than the stuff they try to get us adults to drink. Loaded with broccoli, avocado and flax meal, this smoothie gets its delicious flavor and pretty color from cherries, banana and pomegranate juice.

☐ **Refreshing Watermelon Smoothie**

This smoothie recipe from Live Eat Learn combines the hydrating qualities of watermelon and cucumber with fresh mint to create a delicious smoothie recipes for cancer patientssummertime smoothie. And given the hot weather in Phoenix, this may end up being one of your favorites to whip up year round. Furthermore, since mint is known to help settling stomachs and with other digestive issues, it may be a great option for cancer patients having issues with nausea or indigestion. But be aware, this smoothie is definitely light in the calories department.

☐ **Chocolate Peanut Butter Cup Smoothie**

This smoothie recipe from A Mind Full Mom's blog was inspired by the author's impressive calorie requirements as a result of her cystic fibrosis. However, many cancer patients also struggle to meet their daily calorie quota. This recipe is a delicious, simple way to make headway while ensuring vital nutrients are making up caloric intake. Furthermore, this recipe offers the flexibility of using whole cow's milk or substituting for coconut milk or a favorite nut milk for those with lactose sensitivities. Calling for chia seeds or flax seeds for added fiber, this recipe checks off a lot of boxes on many cancer patients' lists!

☐ Anti-Cancer Green Smoothie Recipe

This anti-cancer smoothie recipe is an evolution of my Power Green Smoothie, but with a special ingredient: frozen broccoli florets.

Broccoli contains sulforaphane, a known anti-cancer food. In this recipe, you actually can't taste the frozen broccoli once it's blended with all of the other great ingredients in this recipe. The fresh ginger, lime juice, and mint leaves are especially important to covering up any of the "green" flavor of the veggies. You have to try it yourself!.

How Broccoli Fights Cancer

Studies show that there are compounds in cruciferous vegetables known as isothiocyanates that fight cancer. However, as far as we know, these compounds are only present in raw or very gently cooked cruciferous vegetables. So, that's why this recipe uses gently blanched and frozen broccoli florets. It's also easier to hide the flavor of frozen broccoli as opposed to fresh broccoli. And, the frozen florets even help to thicken the smoothie.

☐ **Step One**

The first step of this recipe is to gather up your ingredients. The base of the smoothie is made from hemp seeds and water.

☐ Step Two

Combine all of the ingredients in the base of a high-speed blender like a Blendtec or a Vitamix. Blend on high for just about 45 seconds, or until the smoothie is thick and creamy.

☐ Step Three

Divide the smoothie between two glasses and serve immediately. You can store any leftovers in the refrigerator for up to 2 days.

If you're a fan of broccoli, you might also like this easy step-by-step guide for how to sprout broccoli seeds on your countertop without dirt. Sprouting broccoli and eating a tablespoon or two a day is another way to help prevent and fight cancer.

☐ **Best cancer milkshakes ever!!!**

Ingredients

☐ 1 cup milk or nutrition supplement

☐ 2 tablespoons peanut butter

☐ cocoa powder

☐ 1 medium frozen banana

☐ 1 cup fresh spinach or 1/2 to 1 cup frozen spinach

This recipe, it's a great source of protein. It's made all from a variety of plant food, a little bit of milk, you can choose different, your favorite choice, and then it tastes like a chocolate peanut butter milk shake.

☐ So here we have our ingredients.

We have 1 cup of milk, so go ahead and put that in there. I'm going to tell you a little bit about the favorite milk that I recommend. So when you are using milk in your smoothie you want it to be a source of protein, so I would choose a milk that does give you at least 8 grams of protein per cup. Today I'm actually using this particular brand, and they don't even pay me to say it, but it is Fairlife milk. It actually has 15 grams of protein per cup. It is based on cow's milk but does have extra protein and it's also lactose-free, so I use that a lot with fruits when I don't know what kinds of food sensitivities people will have. So we put the milk in.

☐ We put 2 tablespoons of peanut butter.

And my favorite type of peanut butter, I don't have a brand that's my favorite, I just recommend that you look at the ingredient list, and the ingredients should be peanuts, salt, period, end of story. Peanut butter should be peanuts and maybe a little salt for flavoring. So we're putting 2 tablespoons in there, and 2 tablespoons of peanut butter is about 7 grams of protein.

☐ Now, make it chocolatey.

We are using the cocoa powder, and I use a variety of different cocoa powders, but I will say this is my favorite for making things taste really chocolatey.

☐ And then the other two ingredients that you need, first of all a frozen banana.

 So one medium-size frozen banana. I always wait until my bananas go a little bit brown, wait a little bit longer, and then I tear them into pieces and keep them in a freezer-safe container.

☐ The other thing I have here is the spinach, already pre-measured and frozen with the banana.

So you can either use fresh spinach in this recipe, 1 cup of fresh spinach, or you can use anywhere from 1/2 to 1 cup of frozen spinach. So in here I have a cup of frozen spinach, and then I have my one frozen banana. It makes it really convenient if you have them already ready, frozen together so you can just pull them out and pour them in your blender.

My tip, I have had a chef tell me that if you're making smoothies, you want to put the liquid ingredients towards the blade and then the more solid ones above that. There's your smoothie tip. And I'm going to blend it. And there we have it. Kind of the thing that I recommend if you have somebody who is not interested in having a green smoothie with the spinach in it, they're not sure they're going to like it, you can always make it without the spinach. They can taste it. Then make it with the spinach, have them taste it again. A lot of people find out that they like it better with the spinach. And then if you are also somebody going through treatment and needing extra protein or extra calories, you can actually make this recipe using a nutrition supplement drink like Boost or Ensure or whatever store brand in place of the milk, and that adds even more calories and protein. So those are a few different options.

☐ Best Cancer milkshakes ever 2.

Ingredients

☐ 2 cups soy milk

☐ 1 cup orange juice

☐ 1 pound ripe papaya, peeled, pitted, and cubed

☐ 2 bananas, sliced

☐ 2 tablespoons honey

☐ Ice

☐ Sprig of fresh mint, for garnish

Directions

☐ Step 1

Place soy milk, orange juice, papaya, bananas, honey, and ice in the jar of a blender; blend until smooth. Serve garnished with mint.

☐ **Best Cancer milkshakes ever 3.**

Ingredients

☐ 2 cups frozen unsweetened blueberries (do not thaw)

☐ 1/2 cup orange juice (calcium-fortified preferred)

☐ 3/4 cup low-fat or nonfat vanilla yogurt

☐ 1/2 medium frozen banana

☐ 1/2 tsp. pure vanila extract

☐ Makes 2 servings. Per serving: 220 calories, 2.5 g total fat (1 g saturated fat, 0 g trans fat), 5 mg cholesterol, 46 g carbohydrates, 6 g protein, 5 g dietary fiber, 65 mg sodium, 35 g sugar.

Directions

☐ Place blueberries, orange juice, yogurt, banana and vanilla into blender.

☐ Cover securely and blend for 30 to 35 seconds or until thick and smooth. For thinner smoothies, add more juice; for thicker smoothies, add more frozen fruit.

☐ Pour into 2 glasses and serve immediately.

Notes

☐ Don't have frozen blueberries? Try frozen pineapple, cherries or mango.

☐ GINGER GREEN SMOOTHIE

This Ginger Green Smoothie has been a wonderful recipe for many people, thanks to the power of plants (especially ginger root!). So often the nutrients fruit contains aren't used by the body. If the body doesn't have the tools to properly digest, absorb, and eventually use all those great nutrients they go to waste. In this ginger smoothie, nothing the apple brings to the table is wasted thanks to its good friend, ginger. Apples and ginger make the perfect combo in this ginger smoothie recipe. Besides being absolutely delicious, apples and ginger also provide a fantastic combination of health benefits that have been shown to reduce the risk of cancer.

WHY THIS GINGER GREEN SMOOTHIE RAWKS

Apples are considered a cancer-fighting food because of the antioxidants that fight on the front lines against free radicals. Free radicals cause oxidative stress, which damages cells and DNA. These issues open the door for cancer. Apples are able to reduce oxidative stress by eliminating these free radicals. Who knew?! But wait, that's not all! One of the most impressive antioxidants found in apples is quercetin. On top of eliminating free radicals, this antioxidant stops mutating cells from damaging surrounding cells. If cells are not allowed to contaminate one another, cancer can't spread. Apples also contain phenolic compounds, a class of chemical compounds that have been proven to prevent cancer. Phenolic compounds enhance the immune system and assist in preventing the spread of cancerous cells. Talk about a hard-working fruit! Apples provide all these benefits and a ton of vitamins and minerals like vitamin C, potassium, vitamin K, and magnesium.

THE POWER OF GINGER IN THIS GREEN SMOOTHIE

Ginger helps the body make the most of these nutrients by allowing for proper nutrient absorption. This means ginger promotes a healthy digestive system by making sure that nothing gets backed up and everything is put to good use. In addition to helping regulate the metabolism, ginger also promotes a strong immune system because it helps clean out bacteria in the colon. Pair this with all the nutrients found in apples and you can be confident that you are making the most of the nutrients available in your Ginger Smoothie.

GINGER GREEN SMOOTHIE

INGREDIENTS

☐ 1 cup spinach (fresh)

☐ 1 cup almond milk (unsweetened)

☐ 1/2 banana

☐ 1 apple (any variety, core removed)

☐ 1/4 inch ginger (peeled)

INSTRUCTIONS

☐   Blend spinach and almond milk together until smooth.

☐   remaining ingredients and blend again.

NOTES

*Use at least one frozen fruit to make smoothie cold.

☐ **Strawberry Banana Smoothie**

Strawberry and banana puts the smooth in smoothie! There is no better way to describe the blending of tart strawberries and mellow bananas in this recipe. Tasting Guidelines: Taste is sweet. Weight is medium. Texture is smooth. Good for people with low to severe treatment side effects. Cooking for Chemo focuses on teaching you how to make your food taste good again during cancer and chemotherapy treatments. The flavor and cooking techniques contained within our easy to make recipes will help improve your quality of life as you go through cancer and chemotherapy treatments. Strawberry and banana puts the smooth in smoothie! There is no better way to describe the blending of tart strawberries and mellow bananas in this recipe. Tasting Guidelines: Taste is sweet. Weight is medium. Texture is smooth. Good for people with low to severe treatment side effects.

Ingredients

☐ ½ c. milk

- ☐ ¼ c. honey Greek yogurt

- ☐ 5 frozen strawberries

- ☐ 1 ripe banana

- ☐ ½ c. ice cubes

- ☐ 1 scoop chocolate protein powder optional

- ☐ Flavor Balancers

- ☐ 2 tbsp. sugar

Instructions

- ☐ Add all ingredients into the blender and cover.

☐ Activate the blender. If you have frozen ingredients that are not cooperating, use the pulse function and a little finesse to pulse your way into the perfect mixture.

☐ Taste you smoothie and adjust. Is there too much or not enough of a certain ingredient or flavor? Adjust the flavors just like you would do anything else.

☐ Serve in a glass with a straw. Garnish if desired.

Notes

For extra protein and a fun new twist on my favorite smoothie, add chocolate protein powder

☐ **Filling fruit smoothie**

Oats, yoghurt and peanut butter make this smoothie a meal in a glass. Our healthy fruit smoothies are soothing on your throat, suitable for people experiencing mouth problems as a result of cancer treatment. Mouth problems are a common side-effect of cancer, making eating meals a real challenge. This filling and refreshing smoothie is a soothing option. See all our recipes for people living with cancer.This recipe has been designed by Sarah Drabble. It is taken from Eat Well During Cancer, our booklet helping you to cope with the side-effects of cancer.

Ingredients

☐ 100ml whole milk

☐ 1 level tablespoon skimmed milk powder

☐ 1 tablespoon natural yoghurt

☐ Ice cubes (optional)

☐ 1 heaped teaspoon peanut butter (ideally a brand that contains no added salt and sugar)

☐ 1 medium banana

☐ 160g frozen berries

☐ 40g oats

☐ 15g seeds

Time, 5 Minutes, SERVES:2, CALORIES:312, FAT:12.2g, SALT:0.2g, SUGAR:21.1g

Method

☐ Place all the ingredients in a blender, and blend until smooth.

☐ Pour into a glass and serve.

. If you have cancer, eating right can give you strength you need. Smoothies are one way to get the nutrients your body uses to fight the disease and handle the effects of treatment. Smoothies are a good option if your treatment gives you side effects. Smoothies are also cold, which can soothe a sore mouth and throat.